FUNCTIONAL MEDICINE FOR NURSE PRACTITIONERS

A PRACTICAL GUIDE

© **Copyright 2024 - All rights reserved.**

The content contained within this book may not be reproduced, duplicated or transmitted without direct written permission from the author or the publisher.

Under no circumstances will any blame or legal responsibility be held against the publisher, or author, for any damages, reparation, or monetary loss due to the information contained within this book. Either directly or indirectly.

Legal Notice:

This book is copyright protected. This book is only for personal use. You cannot amend, distribute, sell, use, quote or paraphrase any part, or the content within this book, without the consent of the author or publisher.

Disclaimer Notice:

Please note the information contained within this document is for educational and entertainment purposes only. All effort has been executed to present accurate, up to date, and reliable, complete information. No warranties of any kind are declared or implied. Readers acknowledge that the author is not engaging in the rendering of legal, financial, medical or professional advice. The content within this book has been derived from various sources. Please consult a licensed professional before attempting any techniques outlined in this book.

By reading this document, the reader agrees that under no circumstances is the author responsible for any losses, direct or indirect, which are incurred as a result of the use of information contained within this document, including, but not limited to, — errors, omissions, or inaccuracies.

DESCRIPTION 4

INTRODUCTION 7

CHAPTER 1: RETHINKING DISEASE: FROM SYMPTOMS TO ROOT CAUSES 11

CHAPTER 2: THE ART AND SCIENCE OF PATIENT-CENTERED ASSESSMENT 20

CHAPTER 3: MASTERING FUNCTIONAL MEDICINE TOOLS: NUTRITION, SUPPLEMENTS, AND LIFESTYLE 34

CHAPTER 4: CASE-BASED LEARNING: REAL-LIFE SCENARIOS IN FUNCTIONAL MEDICINE 48

CHAPTER 5: BUILDING YOUR PRACTICE: INTEGRATING FUNCTIONAL MEDICINE IN REAL-WORLD SETTINGS 63

CONCLUSION 75

Description

Are you a nurse practitioner ready to elevate your practice and offer patients more than symptom management?

Functional medicine is revolutionizing healthcare by targeting the root causes of illness rather than just treating symptoms. While conventional medicine often addresses isolated issues, functional medicine takes a systems-based approach, viewing the body as interconnected and deeply influenced by lifestyle, environment, and diet. *Functional Medicine for Nurse Practitioners: A Practical Guide* provides the roadmap you need to integrate this powerful, holistic approach into your practice, transforming your patient care and outcomes.

Inside, you'll discover a comprehensive guide designed to empower nurse practitioners to incorporate functional medicine principles seamlessly into their daily routines. This book takes you step-by-step through assessments, treatments, and practical applications, including real-life case studies that demonstrate how functional medicine makes a difference for chronic and complex conditions.

Here's a glimpse of what you'll learn:

- **Foundational Principles of Functional Medicine**: Understand the philosophy of treating patients as whole individuals, identifying the root causes of illness, and working collaboratively with patients for sustained health improvement.

- **Advanced Tools for Patient Assessment**: Learn how to use the Functional Medicine Matrix, patient-centered history-taking, and diagnostics to uncover patterns and connections within your patients' symptoms.

- **Proven Interventions in Functional Medicine**: Explore core interventions that make functional medicine effective, from dietary modifications and targeted supplements to personalized lifestyle adjustments that optimize health outcomes.

- **Real-Life Case Studies**: See functional medicine in action as you walk through patient scenarios for autoimmune conditions, metabolic syndrome, mental health, and more—discovering how to apply principles to get transformative results.

- **Strategies for Integrating Functional Medicine**: Overcome the common challenges of time, resources, and compliance by adopting proven workflows, documentation techniques, and efficient systems that streamline functional medicine into any practice setting.

This practical guide goes beyond theory, equipping you with the actionable tools and insights needed to make functional medicine a sustainable part of your practice. Whether you're new to functional medicine or looking to deepen your expertise, this book will empower you to provide the comprehensive, patient-centered care that today's complex health challenges demand.

Ready to lead the way in transformative patient care? *Functional Medicine for Nurse Practitioners* is your essential guide to building a practice where every patient leaves feeling heard, understood, and truly healed. Don't wait to make functional medicine an impactful part of your career—start your journey to deeper, more effective patient care today!

Introduction

"The greatest medicine of all is teaching people how not to need it."
*– **Hippocrates***

A patient sits before you, describing years of symptoms: fatigue, headaches, digestive discomfort, a nagging sense that something's wrong, but no clear answers in sight. They've cycled through specialists, tests, and medications, finding only temporary relief. Each visit to the clinic becomes a reminder of the limitations of symptom-based treatment. As a nurse practitioner, you're driven to help patients find lasting solutions, but conventional tools feel inadequate for complex, chronic conditions. You know there's a better way—one that addresses the root causes of illness and restores true health. This book is here to help you make that shift.

Functional medicine offers a revolutionary approach to patient care, one that centers on treating the root causes of illness rather than simply managing symptoms. Unlike traditional medicine, which often focuses on isolated symptoms or single-organ systems, functional medicine uses a systems-based approach, recognizing that the body's systems are interconnected and that diet, lifestyle, and environmental factors play critical roles in health. This approach allows for a more thorough, patient-centered model that not only addresses immediate health concerns but also aims to prevent future ones.

For nurse practitioners, this approach aligns closely with the values and strengths of their profession: holistic assessment, patient education, and a commitment to preventive care. Nurse practitioners are well-positioned to adopt functional medicine because of their ability to foster close, empathetic relationships with patients, spending the time necessary to understand each individual's full health picture. This book serves as a practical guide, equipping you with the tools, techniques, and real-world examples needed to seamlessly integrate functional medicine into your practice. It aims to empower you to deliver transformative care for patients, particularly those with chronic and complex conditions, who can benefit most from a root-cause approach.

As healthcare's landscape evolves, nurse practitioners are becoming essential in meeting the rising demand for patient-centered, comprehensive care. With advanced training and a commitment to addressing the whole patient, nurse practitioners often provide care that goes beyond routine symptom management. They typically spend more time with patients, allowing for deeper exploration of health histories, lifestyle factors, and personal goals—elements central to the functional medicine approach.

Functional medicine naturally complements the nurse practitioner's role, which already emphasizes preventive care, health promotion, and patient education. In functional medicine, practitioners work closely with patients to identify the underlying causes of illness, crafting treatment plans that include lifestyle-based solutions, nutrition, and non-pharmaceutical interventions. However, integrating functional medicine into a conventional setting comes with challenges, from time constraints to limited resources. This book will address these barriers, providing strategies and insights to help nurse practitioners overcome them and bring functional medicine principles into daily practice effectively.

This book is structured to provide nurse practitioners with a comprehensive foundation in functional medicine, gradually building skills and knowledge through interconnected sections. Each part focuses on essential elements, from understanding root-cause care and assessment tools to practical interventions and real-world applications. Together, these sections guide you step-by-step, equipping you with a toolkit for integrating functional medicine into your practice effectively.

For best results, treat this book as a practical resource, applying its insights gradually. Take notes, reflect on your current approach, and consider implementing one small change from each section. These incremental steps help translate knowledge into real, transformative practice, allowing you to experience functional medicine's impact firsthand rather than reading passively. The tools and strategies provided are designed for immediate application, supporting you in creating a more patient-centered, holistic practice from the ground up.

Functional medicine invites a shift in mindset, from a conventional, symptom-focused approach to one that seeks the deeper causes of health concerns. This book encourages you to approach it with an openness to rethink established practices, not to replace traditional methods but to expand them. Functional medicine allows nurse practitioners to offer patients a more comprehensive path to health, combining the best of both worlds: the precision of modern medicine with the holistic focus on prevention and root-cause care.

This approach is particularly powerful for chronic conditions, which often demand ongoing management and resilient solutions. By addressing root causes rather than only symptoms, nurse practitioners can reduce the need for repetitive treatments, providing patients with a pathway toward lasting wellness. Functional medicine offers a chance to make a significant difference in the lives of those dealing with persistent, complex health issues, empowering them to take ownership of their health outcomes.

As you move forward, consider yourself a catalyst for change in healthcare. By adopting functional medicine principles, you become part of a vision that emphasizes prevention, education, and patient empowerment, ultimately leading to healthier communities. Nurse practitioners have the potential to transform not only individual lives but also the broader healthcare system, moving toward one that values comprehensive, sustainable health for all.

Chapter 1: Rethinking Disease: From Symptoms to Root Causes

"Healing is a matter of time, but it is sometimes also a matter of opportunity."
– Hippocrates

The same exhausted look crosses her face every time she visits the clinic. A middle-aged woman, Jane has been struggling with relentless fatigue, joint pain, and brain fog. She's seen specialist after specialist, endured countless tests, and left with prescriptions that blunt the pain but never solve it. Her frustration is palpable—each visit, a new doctor, another test, and yet no lasting answers. This is where functional medicine steps in, offering an alternative to the endless cycle of symptom management by addressing what's beneath her symptoms.

In this chapter, we'll explore how functional medicine shifts the focus from simply managing symptoms to identifying and treating underlying causes. Conventional medicine, while vital for acute care, often falls short when dealing with chronic illnesses like Jane's. Nurse practitioners (NPs) will see how functional medicine's root-cause philosophy provides a structured, science-backed approach to treating the entire person. We'll examine the limitations of conventional symptom-focused strategies, delve into the foundational principles of functional medicine, and discuss practical ways NPs can start incorporating these insights to transform patient care.

By understanding how to shift from "What is the symptom?" to "Why is this symptom occurring?" nurse practitioners can offer patients a deeper, more effective level of care that tackles the origins of chronic conditions rather than simply masking them. This chapter will empower NPs to rethink disease, opening up a new, actionable framework that aligns with the demands and complexities of modern healthcare.

1.1 Unmasking the Mystery of Chronic Illness

Conventional medicine is exceptional at acute care—think trauma, infections, or immediate, life-threatening situations. However, when it comes to chronic conditions like autoimmune disorders, irritable bowel syndrome (IBS), or chronic fatigue syndrome, its primary approach often centers on symptom management rather than understanding the full picture. In these cases, patients may receive multiple prescriptions aimed at relieving pain, inflammation, or digestive discomfort, yet these treatments frequently address only the surface level. Symptoms might lessen, but the underlying issues persist, leaving patients in a frustrating cycle where true healing remains out of reach.

Functional medicine, by contrast, aims to identify and address the root causes of disease. Rather than merely prescribing medication to mitigate symptoms, this approach digs deeper to ask *why* these symptoms are manifesting in the first place. In functional medicine, symptoms are seen as clues—signs of underlying imbalances or disruptions in the body's systems that need to be addressed. This doesn't mean ignoring symptoms; rather, it means using them as a guide to look deeper and identify the root issues driving a patient's condition. This approach requires a more holistic perspective that considers the interactions between lifestyle, genetics, and environmental factors.

Several fundamental differences set functional medicine apart from conventional approaches. First, functional medicine views the patient as a whole, interconnected system, rather than focusing on isolated organs or symptoms. Second, it seeks patterns within the body's systems, understanding that symptoms in one area may have roots in another. For example, digestive issues may influence mental health, and vice versa. Finally, functional medicine emphasizes prevention by identifying potential imbalances before they escalate into chronic illness.

Consider the case of a hypothetical patient named Mark, a 45-year-old man struggling with persistent joint pain, digestive issues, and fatigue. Conventional treatment might involve anti-inflammatory medications for the pain and a prescription for acid reflux. However, a functional medicine approach would examine his lifestyle, diet, stress levels, and sleep patterns. Through this analysis, it could become clear that his joint pain and digestive symptoms stem from chronic inflammation due to a poor diet and unaddressed stress. By addressing his nutrition and implementing stress-reduction techniques, Mark's symptoms can improve holistically, targeting the root causes rather than masking symptoms alone.

This shift—from treating individual symptoms to addressing the root cause—empowers nurse practitioners to help patients achieve meaningful, lasting relief and supports a healthcare model focused on wellness, prevention, and long-term health.

1.2 Functional Medicine 101: The Core Principles

Functional medicine is built on foundational principles that diverge from the conventional model, centering around three core ideas: biochemical individuality, dynamic balance, and patient-centered care. Each of these principles underlines the belief that understanding the person behind the symptoms is essential for effective treatment.

Biochemical Individuality

Every individual has a unique genetic makeup that influences how they respond to their environment, lifestyle, and potential treatments. This concept of biochemical individuality acknowledges that genetic and biochemical differences mean that two patients with the same condition may require entirely different approaches to achieve optimal health. For instance, one person's gut may metabolize certain foods or medications differently due to genetic variations affecting their enzyme activity. Recognizing and respecting these differences allows practitioners to tailor treatments more precisely, optimizing health outcomes for each patient based on their specific biological needs.

Dynamic Balance

Health is not simply the absence of disease but the presence of balance among the body's various systems. Dynamic balance emphasizes the interconnected nature of body functions, highlighting that disruptions in one area can impact multiple others. For example, hormonal imbalances might influence immune function or even mental health. Functional medicine practitioners aim to restore this equilibrium, helping the body return to a balanced state. When systems are in harmony, patients experience not just the relief of symptoms but an enhancement in overall well-being.

Patient-Centered Care

Unlike the symptom-focused approach common in conventional medicine, functional medicine places the patient's story, lifestyle, and personal experiences at the heart of diagnosis and treatment. Functional medicine practitioners see each patient as a unique case, taking time to understand the individual's history, lifestyle choices, and environmental exposures. This approach not only helps uncover the root causes of illness but also fosters trust and cooperation, as patients feel seen and heard. It empowers patients to take an active role in their own care, ultimately supporting more effective and sustainable health outcomes.

Overview of Systems Biology

Systems biology underpins the functional medicine approach by viewing the body as an interconnected network rather than isolated parts. Systems biology emphasizes that body systems work in concert, and changes in one system can create ripples across others. One common example is the gut-brain axis: imbalances in gut bacteria can influence mental health, affecting mood, cognition, and stress resilience. Similarly, chronic inflammation in the digestive system may exacerbate joint pain or even contribute to cardiovascular issues. By examining these interconnections, functional medicine practitioners can address health issues in a more comprehensive way.

Why Functional Medicine Works for Chronic Conditions

Chronic conditions like diabetes, autoimmune disorders, and cardiovascular disease often stem from complex, multifactorial origins. Functional medicine's holistic approach to health, with its emphasis on systems thinking and root-cause analysis, is ideally suited to tackle these complexities. Rather than focusing on isolated symptoms, functional medicine assesses a patient's entire health picture, allowing practitioners to develop targeted interventions that address the core drivers of illness. This approach reduces dependency on symptom-focused medications and instead promotes sustainable improvements by addressing the underlying issues directly.

Practical Implications for Nurse Practitioners

For nurse practitioners, adopting these principles transforms the patient care experience. By understanding the nuances of biochemical individuality, they can personalize care that aligns with each patient's unique profile. Systems biology allows them to recognize patterns and relationships across symptoms that might otherwise go unnoticed, providing insights for comprehensive treatment plans. Patient-centered care empowers NPs to connect deeply with their patients, gathering information that can be crucial in pinpointing root causes. As a result, NPs are equipped to provide more holistic, preventative, and lasting healthcare solutions, ultimately leading to better outcomes and greater patient satisfaction.

1.3 Systems Biology: The Foundation of Functional Healing

Defining Systems Biology

Systems biology is the study of the body as an interconnected web of systems rather than isolated organs. In functional medicine, this approach is foundational because it recognizes that a disruption in one area can lead to imbalances in others. Rather than viewing symptoms in isolation, systems biology allows practitioners to identify how a single issue may create a chain reaction of health problems across different bodily systems. This perspective is crucial for addressing chronic conditions, which often involve complex, multifactorial origins that span multiple systems.

Highlighting Interconnected Body Systems

Two major examples illustrate the interconnectedness of body systems and how imbalances in one can lead to issues in others:

- **Gut-Brain Axis**: Research shows that the gut and brain are in constant communication. An imbalance in gut bacteria, for example, can impact neurotransmitter production, influencing mood, stress levels, and cognitive function. This connection is why individuals with gut health issues may also experience symptoms like anxiety, depression, or brain fog.

- **Hormone-Immunity Link**: Hormones play a vital role in immune function. For example, cortisol, the body's primary stress hormone, can suppress immune activity when levels are consistently elevated due to chronic stress. This link explains why hormonal imbalances can weaken the immune system, making individuals more susceptible to infections and inflammation-related conditions.

How Nurse Practitioners Can Use Systems Thinking

Nurse practitioners can incorporate systems thinking into their practice by taking a more comprehensive view of each patient's symptoms. Some practical steps include:

- **Asking Broader Questions**: Instead of focusing solely on the primary complaint, NPs can inquire about a wide range of symptoms, lifestyle habits, and environmental factors that might be contributing to the patient's condition.

- **Looking for Patterns**: Identifying patterns across seemingly unrelated symptoms—like digestive issues and anxiety—can reveal underlying connections between body systems that may otherwise be missed.

By embracing systems biology, NPs can develop more targeted and effective treatment strategies that address the root causes of health issues, leading to better patient outcomes and a more integrative approach to care.

Key Takeaways

- Functional medicine emphasizes identifying and addressing the root causes of illness rather than focusing solely on symptoms.

- Systems biology provides a framework for understanding how imbalances in one area can impact other body systems.

- The principles of functional medicine enable nurse practitioners to adopt a personalized, patient-centered approach to healthcare.

- Applying systems thinking can improve outcomes in chronic condition management by recognizing interconnected symptoms and underlying causes.

Take a moment to consider one patient in your practice who has persistent, complex symptoms—perhaps a patient with recurring digestive issues and anxiety, or chronic fatigue with no clear origin. Reflect on how a root-cause approach might help uncover connections between symptoms and underlying imbalances. Start thinking about potential links between body systems that may be contributing to the patient's condition. In the next chapter, we'll explore patient-centered assessments, equipping you with tools to gather and interpret these insights effectively.

Chapter 2: The Art and Science of Patient-Centered Assessment

"The good physician treats the disease; the great physician treats the patient who has the disease."
— William Osler

The woman in front of you complains of migraines, constant fatigue, and digestive problems, issues she's been managing with various specialists over the years. Each symptom has been addressed individually, yet nothing seems to provide lasting relief. No clear diagnosis ties it all together, leaving her frustrated and searching for answers. It's cases like these where a comprehensive, patient-centered assessment can make a profound difference. By stepping back and considering all aspects of her health—her lifestyle, environment, stress levels, and genetic predispositions—a clearer picture emerges, often revealing the interconnected factors driving her symptoms.

This chapter introduces the tools and techniques essential for effective patient-centered assessment in functional medicine. First, we'll explore the Functional Medicine Matrix, a powerful framework that helps practitioners view patients holistically and recognize connections across symptoms and body systems. Next, we'll cover advanced patient history-taking methods, emphasizing how thorough and strategic questioning can uncover lifestyle, environmental, and genetic influences often overlooked. Finally, we'll discuss advanced diagnostics that go beyond standard testing to provide a deeper, more nuanced understanding of the body's internal state.

Equipped with these tools, nurse practitioners will gain the skills needed to assess patients more thoroughly, identifying root causes with greater precision and setting the stage for more effective treatment plans.

2.1 The Functional Medicine Matrix: Seeing the Patient as a Whole

Functional medicine emphasizes that each patient is more than a collection of symptoms—they are a complex, interconnected system. The Functional Medicine Matrix is a tool designed to help practitioners organize and analyze patient information in a holistic way, visualizing how various symptoms, lifestyle factors, and body systems interact. By using this matrix, nurse practitioners can shift from a symptom-focused approach to one that seeks connections and root causes, enabling them to develop targeted, effective treatment plans that address underlying issues rather than just surface-level symptoms.

Introducing the Functional Medicine Matrix

The Functional Medicine Matrix is a structured tool that organizes information across multiple domains of a patient's health. It highlights patterns and connections among symptoms, lifestyle factors, genetic predispositions, and clinical imbalances. This matrix allows practitioners to systematically assess how various factors influence each other within a patient's body. By visualizing these interactions, nurse practitioners can identify key areas where intervention may have the greatest impact on overall health.

Matrix Components

1. **Antecedents, Triggers, and Mediators (ATMs)**

- **Antecedents** are factors that predispose a person to health issues. This includes genetics, early-life exposures, and family history. Knowing a patient's antecedents provides context about their risk for specific conditions.

- **Triggers** are events or exposures that provoke symptoms or exacerbate conditions. These may include infections, physical or emotional trauma, dietary changes, or environmental toxins.

- **Mediators** are factors that sustain or worsen health issues over time, such as chronic inflammation or oxidative stress. Identifying these helps practitioners focus on the ongoing influences that contribute to a patient's symptoms.

Together, ATMs help practitioners map out a patient's health timeline and understand how past events and ongoing factors contribute to their current condition.

2. Modifiable Lifestyle Factors

This section assesses lifestyle elements that patients can actively change. Key areas include:

- **Diet**: Nutritional intake, food sensitivities, and eating patterns.

- **Stress**: Levels of chronic stress and stress management practices.

- **Sleep**: Quality, quantity, and consistency of sleep.

- **Exercise and Movement**: Physical activity habits, including frequency, type, and intensity.

- **Relationships and Social Support**: The influence of relationships and social interactions on mental and emotional health.

Modifiable lifestyle factors are essential because they offer practical starting points for intervention. Small changes in these areas can significantly improve health outcomes, especially when they address underlying imbalances identified in the Matrix.

3. **Core Clinical Imbalances**

The Matrix also focuses on identifying physiological imbalances that may contribute to illness, such as:

- **Inflammation and Immune Dysregulation**: Chronic inflammation and immune response issues that may drive conditions like autoimmune diseases.

- **Detoxification and Biotransformation**: How the body processes and removes toxins.

- **Hormone and Neurotransmitter Balance**: Levels and interactions of hormones and neurotransmitters affecting mood, energy, and metabolism.

- o **Energy Production**: Mitochondrial function and energy levels, often impacting fatigue and metabolic health.

- o **Digestive Function and Microbiome Health**: Digestive efficiency, nutrient absorption, and microbiome balance.

By identifying these imbalances, practitioners can develop a focused treatment approach that targets the fundamental physiological processes contributing to the patient's symptoms.

How to Use the Matrix in Practice

Using the Functional Medicine Matrix begins with a thorough collection of patient data across these categories. Nurse practitioners can:

- **Organize Patient Information**: Categorize symptoms, lifestyle habits, and medical history within the Matrix structure, allowing for a comprehensive view of the patient's health.

- **Identify Patterns**: Look for patterns and connections that traditional models may overlook, such as the link between dietary habits and chronic inflammation.

- **Set Priorities**: Determine which areas, such as reducing inflammation or addressing hormonal imbalances, should be prioritized for intervention based on their influence on other systems.

The Matrix allows practitioners to construct a more precise and individualized treatment plan by focusing on the interactions among various health factors rather than isolating symptoms.

Case Example

Consider a patient named Sarah, a 52-year-old woman experiencing chronic migraines, fatigue, and digestive issues. A conventional approach might treat each symptom separately with medications for pain, energy, and digestion. However, when mapped onto the Functional Medicine Matrix, Sarah's symptoms reveal clear patterns. Her antecedents include a family history of autoimmune conditions, and her triggers include a period of high work stress. Her lifestyle shows minimal physical activity, irregular sleep, and a diet high in processed foods. Core clinical imbalances highlight chronic inflammation and hormonal dysregulation.

This mapping process reveals that her migraines and fatigue may stem largely from inflammation and dietary factors rather than isolated neurological issues. By focusing on dietary adjustments, stress reduction, and supporting hormone balance, Sarah's treatment plan addresses the root causes of her symptoms, leading to improvements in multiple areas of her health simultaneously. The Functional Medicine Matrix thus transforms a complex presentation into a targeted, effective strategy for long-term relief.

2.2 Comprehensive History Taking: The Story Behind Symptoms

A thorough patient history is the cornerstone of functional medicine, offering insights that are often missed in a symptom-focused approach. Functional medicine relies on understanding a patient's unique background, lifestyle, and environmental exposures to identify root causes and hidden connections. By constructing a detailed health narrative, nurse practitioners can gather invaluable information that points toward effective, personalized treatment plans.

Importance of Patient History

In functional medicine, a patient's story isn't just background information—it's a critical part of diagnosis. Chronic symptoms often stem from a combination of genetic, lifestyle, and environmental factors that interact over time. A comprehensive history allows practitioners to uncover these layers, revealing patterns and connections that help pinpoint underlying causes. For example, a patient's stressors, diet, and exposure to toxins may all contribute to their chronic inflammation. By understanding the full picture, practitioners are better equipped to develop treatment plans that target the roots of illness rather than just its manifestations.

Key Areas to Cover in History Taking

A functional medicine history covers several key areas that collectively provide a detailed view of a patient's health and life circumstances. Each of these components contributes vital clues for developing a root-cause-based treatment approach.

- **Genetics**: Genetic predispositions often shape how a patient responds to their environment and lifestyle. Ask about family history, focusing on chronic conditions that run in the family, such as autoimmune diseases, cardiovascular issues, or mental health disorders. A family history of these conditions may indicate genetic vulnerabilities that can help guide preventive and therapeutic strategies. For example, understanding that a patient has a family history of diabetes may highlight the importance of diet and exercise in managing their blood sugar.

- **Lifestyle**: Lifestyle factors include daily routines, diet, physical activity, and stress management practices. These aspects are foundational to health and can either contribute to or protect against chronic illness. Inquire about the patient's eating habits, exercise routines, and stress levels, as well as their sleep quality and duration. A pattern of poor diet combined with high stress and lack of physical activity may contribute to a range of issues, from hormonal imbalances to digestive dysfunctions.

- **Environment**: Environmental exposures significantly affect health, particularly in patients with chronic conditions. Explore the patient's work environment, home surroundings, and potential exposure to toxins, pollutants, or allergens. A patient who works in a high-stress, industrial setting may be exposed to harmful chemicals or pollutants that contribute to respiratory issues or exacerbate existing inflammatory conditions. Additionally, home environment factors like mold, allergens, or noise pollution can impact a patient's overall well-being.

- **Previous Medical History**: Past illnesses, surgeries, and treatments provide context for the patient's current health challenges. Ask about any previous diagnoses, medications, surgeries, or hospitalizations. Understanding a patient's medical history can shed light on factors that may have contributed to their current condition, such as antibiotic use that affected gut health or surgeries that impacted hormonal balance.

Techniques for Eliciting Detailed Histories

To gather a complete history, practitioners need to create a space where patients feel comfortable sharing openly. Techniques like motivational interviewing and open-ended questioning can help patients reveal key details about their health and lifestyle.

- **Motivational Interviewing**: This technique encourages patients to talk about their health experiences and behaviors, fostering trust and rapport. Asking questions that help patients reflect on their lifestyle choices can reveal insights into behaviors that may be impacting their health. For instance, asking, "What do you think could be affecting your energy levels?" allows patients to explore potential stressors or habits they might not initially consider relevant.

- **Open-Ended Questions**: Questions that invite elaboration, rather than simple yes-or-no answers, help uncover deeper insights into a patient's life. Examples include:

    o "Can you describe a typical day for you?"

- o "What do you find most challenging about managing your health?"

- o "How do you feel your diet and sleep have changed over the past year?"

These questions can reveal lifestyle, emotional, or environmental factors contributing to a patient's condition. For example, a patient mentioning that they often skip meals and struggle with sleep due to work stress offers a glimpse into patterns that may contribute to digestive and metabolic issues.

How to Record and Organize Patient Histories

Documentation is key to making the most of comprehensive histories. Organized records help practitioners identify patterns over time and reference past details quickly and efficiently. Digital tools, such as electronic health records (EHRs) tailored for functional medicine, can streamline this process by providing templates for structured data entry.

- **Use Templates and Checklists**: Structured templates for functional medicine history taking can help ensure all critical areas are covered. Templates allow practitioners to consistently ask about genetics, lifestyle, environment, and medical history in an organized way.

- **Digital Tools for Pattern Recognition**: Digital records enable practitioners to track changes in symptoms, lifestyle factors, and lab results over time, making it easier to recognize patterns that emerge. For instance, a pattern of recurring digestive issues after periods of high stress might prompt targeted interventions, such as stress management strategies or dietary adjustments.

- **Summarize and Synthesize Key Points**: After taking the history, organize the information in a way that highlights key patterns and connections. Summarizing the main antecedents, triggers, and lifestyle factors contributing to the patient's current symptoms provides a clear starting point for treatment.

Example of a Patient History

Consider a patient named Tom, a 40-year-old man experiencing frequent headaches, chronic fatigue, and digestive discomfort. Traditional approaches might treat these symptoms separately with pain relievers and antacids. However, a comprehensive history reveals a different story. Tom reports a family history of autoimmune disease, a high-stress job in a factory setting, frequent junk food meals due to his irregular hours, and exposure to pollutants in his workplace.

By organizing Tom's information using a functional medicine framework, several connections emerge. His family history of autoimmune disease and his high-stress environment point to genetic and environmental factors that could be contributing to inflammation. His diet, low in nutrients and high in processed foods, exacerbates his digestive issues and likely contributes to his fatigue. Additionally, his exposure to pollutants may be increasing his toxic load, placing stress on his liver and contributing to his overall symptoms.

Using this well-organized history, a treatment plan for Tom might focus on:

- Improving his diet by adding nutrient-dense foods to reduce inflammation and support energy levels.

- Implementing stress-reduction practices, such as mindfulness exercises, to mitigate his work-related stress.

- Supporting detoxification with lifestyle changes and supplements to address his exposure to environmental toxins.

Through this approach, Tom's treatment targets the underlying factors rather than merely managing his symptoms. Comprehensive history taking thus enables practitioners to design individualized, effective care plans rooted in an understanding of each patient's unique health landscape.

2.3 Beyond Bloodwork: Advanced Testing for Better Insights

Functional medicine often employs advanced diagnostic tests that go beyond standard bloodwork to provide a comprehensive view of a patient's internal health. These tests are invaluable in uncovering hidden imbalances, giving a more detailed picture of body systems and their interconnections. By examining aspects like gut health, hormone levels, and toxin exposure, nurse practitioners can pinpoint root causes more precisely, creating a tailored treatment plan that addresses the full scope of a patient's condition.

Types of Advanced Tests

- **Gut Health Testing**: This includes microbiome analysis and digestive function tests, which reveal imbalances in gut bacteria and digestive efficiency. Poor gut health is often linked to chronic conditions, from autoimmune disorders to mental health issues.

- **Hormone Testing**: Advanced hormone testing assesses levels of cortisol, thyroid hormones, and sex hormones. Imbalances here can affect everything from energy levels and metabolism to mood and immune function.

- **Nutritional and Toxic Element Testing**: Micronutrient testing measures vitamins, minerals, and antioxidants to identify deficiencies, while toxic element testing detects heavy metals and other toxins. These results provide insight into nutritional gaps and environmental toxin exposure, both of which can drive chronic symptoms.

Interpreting Results for Root Causes

Advanced diagnostics should be interpreted as part of a bigger picture, considering patient history, lifestyle, and other clinical observations. Rather than viewing test results in isolation, practitioners can use them as clues to uncover underlying issues across body systems. For example, low thyroid hormone levels might signal underlying gut health or nutrient absorption issues that also require attention.

When and How to Use These Tests in Practice

Selecting advanced tests should be based on specific symptoms and a thorough patient history. Educate patients on the benefits of these tests, explaining how they contribute to a targeted treatment plan by illuminating deeper imbalances. Transparent communication fosters patient understanding and engagement in their healthcare process.

Key Takeaways

- The Functional Medicine Matrix provides a holistic view of patient health.

- A comprehensive patient history often reveals root causes of chronic symptoms.

- Advanced diagnostics offer insights that standard tests may miss, enabling more precise interventions.

Consider incorporating a comprehensive patient history questionnaire and familiarize yourself with the Functional Medicine Matrix. Reflect on patients in your practice who may benefit from advanced testing to uncover hidden health issues, setting the stage for the next chapter on therapeutic interventions.

Chapter 3: Mastering Functional Medicine Tools: Nutrition, Supplements, and Lifestyle

"Let food be thy medicine, and medicine be thy food."
– Hippocrates

Maria, a 38-year-old patient, had been grappling with chronic fatigue for years. Every day felt like an uphill battle, and she struggled to stay alert and engaged at work. After countless consultations and conventional treatments, she finally began to see change through targeted dietary adjustments, supplements, and lifestyle modifications. By cutting out processed foods, adding nutrient-dense meals, and supporting her body with essential supplements, Maria's energy and focus began to improve noticeably. Over time, with additional lifestyle changes to improve sleep and reduce stress, her fatigue lifted, transforming her day-to-day experience and making a lasting impact on her health.

This chapter covers the core tools of functional medicine that can drive profound change in cases like Maria's. We'll start with the role of functional nutrition, outlining dietary approaches that can address inflammation, balance blood sugar, and improve digestive health. Next, we'll look at supplements and botanicals, including guidelines for choosing high-quality options and tailoring them to individual needs. Finally, we'll explore lifestyle modifications, focusing on sleep, stress management, and physical activity—essential elements that lay the foundation for sustained health improvements. Together, these tools offer nurse practitioners a practical framework to address root causes and support their patients' path to wellness.

3.1 Nourish to Heal: The Transformative Power of Diet

Nutrition is foundational in functional medicine, offering a way to address chronic conditions directly and support overall health at a cellular level. Every patient's nutritional needs are influenced by their unique biochemistry, genetics, lifestyle, and health status. A personalized dietary approach allows nurse practitioners to target specific health issues—such as inflammation, hormonal imbalances, and metabolic dysfunction—by supporting the body with nutrients tailored to each individual. Functional medicine nutrition goes beyond general dietary advice; it's about identifying the foods and nutrients that work best for each patient's needs, providing a powerful tool for managing and even reversing chronic conditions.

Key Dietary Approaches in Functional Medicine

In functional medicine, there are several core dietary approaches that address the root causes of chronic health issues and promote healing:

- **Anti-Inflammatory Diet**: Chronic inflammation is at the heart of many health problems, from autoimmune diseases to cardiovascular issues. An anti-inflammatory diet focuses on whole, unprocessed foods rich in antioxidants, fiber, and healthy fats. Patients are encouraged to eat vegetables, fruits, fatty fish, nuts, seeds, and olive oil while avoiding processed foods, refined sugars, and trans fats. By reducing inflammatory triggers, this diet helps calm the immune system and allows the body to focus on repair and restoration.

- **Elimination Diet**: Food sensitivities can often exacerbate symptoms, such as digestive distress, headaches, skin issues, and fatigue. An elimination diet helps identify which foods may be causing these reactions by systematically removing potential allergens—such as dairy, gluten, soy, and certain nuts—from the patient's diet, then reintroducing them one by one to monitor for adverse reactions. This method allows patients to pinpoint and avoid foods that don't work well with their bodies, providing relief from persistent symptoms.

- **Blood Sugar Balancing**: For patients with energy crashes, mood swings, and cravings, blood sugar balancing is essential. A diet that stabilizes blood sugar focuses on low-glycemic foods, high-quality protein, healthy fats, and fiber. Encouraging patients to eat regular meals that include protein, fiber, and healthy fats helps prevent the spikes and crashes associated with blood sugar fluctuations. This approach not only supports energy and mood but also reduces stress on the pancreas, helping to prevent metabolic disorders like type 2 diabetes.

Practical Tips for Patient Nutrition Counseling

Working with patients to make dietary changes requires practical, achievable strategies that fit their lives and health goals.

- **Goal Setting**: Encourage patients to set realistic, measurable goals. For example, instead of an overwhelming goal like "overhaul my diet," a patient might start with "add one serving of vegetables to each meal." Gradual goals create a sustainable pathway to change and prevent patients from feeling discouraged.

- **Education**: Teaching patients the basics of whole foods versus processed foods can be a game-changer. Explain the health benefits of choosing foods with minimal processing and how these choices impact energy, inflammation, and digestion. Demonstrate how to read food labels to identify hidden sugars, preservatives, and unhealthy fats, empowering patients to make informed choices.

- **Meal Planning**: Practical tips for meal planning and preparation make a new diet easier to implement. Suggest batch cooking on weekends or preparing easy-to-freeze meals, such as vegetable soups, stews, and protein-rich casseroles. For patients with busy schedules, providing ideas for quick, nutritious meals helps them stay on track without feeling overwhelmed.

Case Example

Consider a patient named John, a 45-year-old man with frequent bloating, gas, and fatigue. Despite trying various medications for digestive issues, his symptoms persist. Through a functional medicine approach, John was guided to try an elimination diet to identify potential trigger foods. After removing dairy and gluten for a few weeks, he noticed significant relief in his symptoms. When he reintroduced dairy, his bloating returned, indicating a sensitivity. John also incorporated nutrient-dense foods, including leafy greens, lean proteins, and healthy fats, which provided steady energy throughout the day. Over time, these dietary changes helped not only his digestion but also his energy levels, allowing him to feel better without relying on medication.

Overcoming Common Barriers to Dietary Change

Changing dietary habits can be challenging, especially when patients face obstacles like time constraints, budget limitations, and specific food preferences. Here are some strategies nurse practitioners can use to help patients navigate these challenges effectively:

- **Time Constraints**: Many patients struggle to find time for meal preparation. Suggest batch cooking, where meals can be prepared in large quantities and stored for easy access throughout the week. Recommend healthy, quick options like smoothies with vegetables and protein powder, or salads with pre-washed greens and ready-to-go protein sources like hard-boiled eggs or canned salmon.

- **Budget-Friendly Choices**: Healthy eating doesn't have to be expensive. Encourage patients to shop for seasonal produce and buy in bulk, especially for staple foods like grains, beans, and nuts. Frozen fruits and vegetables are also a cost-effective option that retains high nutritional value.

Providing a list of budget-friendly nutrient-dense foods, like sweet potatoes, brown rice, beans, and leafy greens, can make it easier for patients to eat healthily without breaking the bank.

- **Food Preferences and Cultural Factors**: Respecting patients' cultural backgrounds and food preferences is essential for a successful dietary plan. Work with patients to identify healthy options that align with their traditional diets and tastes. For example, if a patient prefers Mediterranean-style meals, suggest options that incorporate olive oil, fish, legumes, and plenty of vegetables. Personalized nutrition counseling increases adherence and supports long-term dietary changes.

Dietary changes can significantly impact a patient's health, and functional medicine provides a framework that respects each patient's unique biochemistry and lifestyle. Through targeted nutrition counseling and a personalized dietary approach, nurse practitioners can help patients address chronic conditions and support lasting health improvements.

3.2 Supplements and Botanicals: Precision Tools for Healing

Supplements and botanicals can play a vital role in functional medicine, providing targeted support for patients dealing with specific health concerns. While whole foods remain the foundation of any health-focused diet, certain nutrients and compounds may be challenging to obtain in sufficient amounts from food alone, especially for those with unique nutritional needs or chronic conditions. Supplements offer a way to address these gaps, but they must be selected thoughtfully and tailored to each individual's condition, avoiding a one-size-fits-all approach. When used strategically, supplements and botanicals enhance the body's ability to heal, reduce inflammation, and support overall resilience.

Commonly Recommended Supplements in Functional Medicine

Functional medicine practitioners often use specific categories of supplements to target underlying imbalances. Here are a few of the most commonly recommended:

- **Probiotics and Prebiotics**: Gut health is central to overall health, impacting digestion, immune function, and even mood. Probiotics—beneficial bacteria found in supplements—can help restore microbial balance in the gut, especially after antibiotic use or with digestive complaints. Prebiotics, non-digestible fibers that feed beneficial bacteria, support long-term microbiome health. Together, they enhance digestive health and contribute to a balanced gut environment.

- **Anti-Inflammatory Supplements**: Chronic inflammation is a common underlying factor in many health conditions, including autoimmune disorders and cardiovascular issues. Omega-3 fatty acids (found in fish oil) and curcumin (derived from turmeric) are two well-researched anti-inflammatory supplements that can help reduce inflammation at the cellular level. Omega-3s support heart health and brain function, while curcumin offers anti-inflammatory benefits that support joint and immune health.

- **Adaptogens**: Adaptogenic herbs, such as ashwagandha, rhodiola, and holy basil, help the body adapt to and recover from stress by modulating the stress response. Ashwagandha, for instance, has been shown to reduce cortisol levels, which can alleviate symptoms of chronic stress and improve energy. These botanicals are especially beneficial for patients experiencing burnout or adrenal fatigue.

- **Vitamins and Minerals**: Certain vitamins and minerals are often deficient in individuals with chronic health issues. Vitamin D, magnesium, and B vitamins are among the most commonly needed. Vitamin D supports immune function and bone health, while magnesium plays a role in muscle relaxation, sleep, and stress management. B vitamins, particularly B12 and folate, are crucial for energy production, cognitive function, and red blood cell formation.

Guidelines for Selecting and Dosing Supplements

When choosing supplements, quality, dosage, and safety are critical factors to consider. Here are some practical guidelines:

- **Choose High-Quality Supplements**: Not all supplements are created equal. Look for reputable brands that undergo third-party testing for purity and potency. Supplements should be free from artificial fillers, preservatives, and allergens whenever possible. Nurse practitioners can recommend pharmaceutical-grade supplements, ensuring patients receive reliable products.

- **Tailor Dosing to Individual Needs**: Dosage should be based on the patient's specific health condition, age, weight, and overall nutrient status. For example, someone with severe vitamin D deficiency may need higher doses temporarily, followed by maintenance doses. Regular monitoring of nutrient levels through blood tests can guide appropriate adjustments.

- **Safety and Interactions**: Supplements should be selected with an understanding of potential interactions with medications. For instance, omega-3s can thin the blood, so patients on blood-thinning medication should use caution. A thorough patient history can help identify any contraindications and reduce the risk of adverse effects.

Patient Education on Supplements

Educating patients about supplements is essential for ensuring safe and effective use. Here are key points to cover:

- **Consistency**: Explain that regular use is necessary for supplements to be effective. Nutritional deficiencies and chronic conditions develop over time, so patients should commit to a consistent regimen for several weeks or months before expecting significant improvements.

- **Safety**: Encourage patients to adhere to recommended dosages and caution against "doubling up" if they miss a dose. Educate them on possible side effects and interactions, especially if they're taking multiple supplements or prescription medications.

- **Realistic Expectations**: Supplements should be viewed as part of a broader health strategy, not as quick fixes. Reinforce that while supplements can provide valuable support, lasting health improvements often require dietary and lifestyle changes as well.

Case Example

Consider Sarah, a 32-year-old patient struggling with persistent fatigue, brain fog, and stress. After evaluating her lifestyle, lab results, and overall health, her practitioner recommended a targeted regimen including B-complex vitamins, magnesium, and ashwagandha. The B vitamins helped boost her energy by supporting mitochondrial function, while magnesium improved her sleep quality and stress tolerance. Ashwagandha helped her manage stress better, lowering her cortisol levels and improving her energy throughout the day. After three months on this regimen, Sarah reported increased focus, better energy levels, and less tension, allowing her to fully engage in her daily activities. This tailored approach highlights how specific, well-chosen supplements can significantly enhance patient outcomes when combined with lifestyle adjustments and dietary improvements.

3.3 Lifestyle Prescriptions: Sleep, Stress, and Movement

Lifestyle prescriptions are intentional, evidence-based changes to daily habits that support healing and enhance quality of life. In functional medicine, sleep, stress management, and physical activity are considered foundational to overall health. Unlike medications, these lifestyle interventions create sustainable changes that help prevent and manage chronic conditions, making them a vital component of any therapeutic plan. Optimizing these areas supports the body's natural healing processes, helping patients achieve better outcomes and resilience against stressors.

Sleep Optimization

Quality sleep is essential for immune function, cognitive performance, and emotional balance. Here are practical strategies for helping patients improve sleep:

- **Consistent Schedule**: Encourage patients to go to bed and wake up at the same time each day, even on weekends, to regulate their internal clock.

- **Limit Screen Time**: Blue light from phones, computers, and televisions can interfere with melatonin production. Advise patients to avoid screens at least one hour before bed or use blue light filters.

- **Create a Calming Routine**: Suggest a wind-down routine that includes relaxing activities like reading, light stretching, or warm baths to signal to the body that it's time to sleep.

Stress Management Techniques

Effective stress management is crucial, as chronic stress can exacerbate many health conditions. Nurse practitioners can recommend simple, accessible methods for managing stress:

- **Mindfulness and Meditation**: Brief mindfulness exercises or meditation help patients focus on the present moment, reducing anxiety and promoting mental clarity. Starting with just five minutes per day can make a noticeable difference.

- **Breathing Exercises**: Techniques like deep breathing or the "4-7-8" breathing method can calm the nervous system, reducing cortisol levels and promoting relaxation.

Encouraging Movement and Physical Activity

Regular physical activity supports cardiovascular health, improves mood, and boosts energy levels. To make movement accessible for patients of all fitness levels:

- **Short Walks**: Recommend starting with short, daily walks that can be gradually extended. Walking outdoors can enhance mood and reduce stress.

- **Gentle Stretching**: Simple stretching routines, especially in the morning or before bed, improve flexibility and can ease tension.

- **At-Home Exercises**: Suggest easy-to-do exercises like bodyweight squats, lunges, or yoga poses that don't require equipment, making physical activity achievable at home.

Supporting Patient Adherence to Lifestyle Changes

Adopting new habits can be challenging, so helping patients build sustainable routines is essential for long-term success. Effective strategies include:

- **Setting Small Goals**: Encourage patients to set realistic, incremental goals, such as adding one additional hour of sleep or five minutes of exercise each day.

- **Tracking Progress**: Using a journal or app to track improvements in sleep, stress levels, and physical activity can reinforce positive changes and provide a sense of accomplishment.

- **Celebrating Improvements**: Recognize even small victories, as celebrating progress helps maintain motivation and reinforces commitment to lifestyle changes.

Key Takeaways

- Nutrition is foundational in functional medicine and can address root causes.

- Supplements and botanicals provide targeted support for healing.

- Lifestyle modifications in sleep, stress, and movement are essential for long-term health.

Encourage readers to introduce one dietary or lifestyle change in their next patient visit. Suggest identifying a relevant supplement category for common conditions. Prompt readers to consider how these foundational tools will support the more complex case studies discussed in the following chapter.

Chapter 4: Case-Based Learning: Real-Life Scenarios in Functional Medicine

"The good physician treats the disease; the great physician treats the patient who has the disease."
— **William Osler**

Lisa was frustrated. After years of enduring joint pain, constant fatigue, and digestive issues, she'd seen countless specialists and tried various medications. Each appointment focused on managing her symptoms, but no treatment seemed to address her underlying health issues. Then, with a functional medicine approach that focused on identifying root causes, her health finally started to shift. Her practitioner assessed her gut health, inflammation levels, and potential environmental triggers, uncovering patterns that connected her symptoms in a way traditional treatments had missed. With personalized changes in her diet, supplements, and lifestyle, Lisa began to experience real, lasting relief.

This chapter delves into real-life case studies to show how functional medicine principles transform complex, chronic conditions. We'll examine three detailed scenarios—autoimmune conditions, metabolic syndrome, and mental health—each illustrating specific functional tools and approaches in practice. Through these examples, nurse practitioners can see the Functional Medicine Matrix, advanced diagnostics, and lifestyle interventions in action, and understand how addressing root causes leads to more effective, sustainable patient outcomes.

4.1 Autoimmune Mysteries: Unraveling the Immune Response

Autoimmune conditions present a complex challenge, as they often involve persistent inflammation, immune dysregulation, and a variety of symptoms that can affect multiple systems. Functional medicine addresses these conditions by exploring the root causes of immune dysfunction, such as diet, environmental exposures, and lifestyle factors. This approach enables practitioners to develop individualized treatment plans that target underlying imbalances rather than merely suppressing symptoms. In this case study, we'll follow a hypothetical patient with Hashimoto's thyroiditis to illustrate how functional medicine principles can improve outcomes in autoimmune disease.

4.1.1 Patient Background and Symptoms

Emily, a 42-year-old woman, has been struggling with fatigue, joint pain, and digestive issues for over a year. She was recently diagnosed with Hashimoto's thyroiditis, an autoimmune condition that affects thyroid function. Despite taking prescribed thyroid medication, her symptoms persist, impacting her ability to work and engage in daily activities. She also reports frequent bloating, irregular bowel movements, and episodes of brain fog, which she attributes to her thyroid disorder.

Emily's family history reveals that both her mother and aunt have rheumatoid arthritis, suggesting a genetic predisposition to autoimmune conditions. Her lifestyle is high-stress due to a demanding job, and she often skips meals, relying on processed snacks and caffeine to get through the day. Her sleep quality is poor, and she typically feels "wired but tired" at night. Emily's health history shows multiple rounds of antibiotics for recurrent infections in her twenties, which may have disrupted her gut microbiome, potentially influencing her current condition.

4.1.2 Functional Medicine Assessment

Using the Functional Medicine Matrix, Emily's practitioner organizes her case to explore the interconnected factors contributing to her condition. The assessment focuses on identifying antecedents, triggers, and mediators, along with advanced testing to clarify underlying issues.

- **Antecedents**: Emily's family history of autoimmune disease and her history of antibiotic use are significant antecedents. The genetic predisposition, combined with microbiome disruption from antibiotics, suggests an increased risk of immune dysregulation.

- **Triggers**: Key triggers for Emily's condition likely include her high-stress lifestyle, poor diet, and disrupted sleep patterns. Stress can exacerbate immune imbalances and increase inflammation, and inadequate sleep can impair the body's ability to repair and regulate immune function. Her reliance on processed foods and frequent caffeine intake can further drive inflammation and blood sugar instability.

- **Mediators**: Chronic inflammation and poor gut health serve as ongoing mediators, sustaining Emily's symptoms and immune dysregulation. Gut health testing, such as a comprehensive stool analysis, reveals an imbalance in her gut microbiome with low levels of beneficial bacteria and elevated inflammatory markers. Blood tests show increased levels of thyroid antibodies and elevated C-reactive protein (CRP), indicating systemic inflammation. These findings confirm that both gut health and inflammation are central issues in her case.

Advanced testing provides additional insights into her immune function and nutrient status. Tests reveal deficiencies in vitamin D and magnesium, both crucial for immune modulation and inflammatory control. This information allows the practitioner to develop a targeted plan addressing Emily's unique needs.

4.1.3 Developing the Treatment Plan

Emily's treatment plan focuses on reducing inflammation, improving gut health, and supporting her immune system with targeted nutrition and lifestyle changes. The approach is comprehensive, addressing dietary, supplemental, and lifestyle aspects to create a well-rounded intervention.

- **Dietary Changes**: Emily begins an anti-inflammatory diet that emphasizes whole foods rich in antioxidants, fiber, and healthy fats. Her practitioner recommends incorporating foods like leafy greens, fatty fish, berries, and olive oil to reduce inflammation. Additionally, she starts an elimination diet, temporarily removing gluten and dairy—common triggers for individuals with autoimmune conditions. After several weeks, she'll reintroduce these foods individually to assess their impact on her symptoms.

- **Supplements**: The supplementation plan includes vitamin D and magnesium to address her deficiencies, with omega-3 fatty acids (from fish oil) and turmeric (curcumin) to provide further anti-inflammatory support. Probiotics and prebiotics are introduced to restore balance in her gut microbiome, along with glutamine to support gut lining integrity. For thyroid support, her practitioner recommends selenium and zinc, minerals that play a role in thyroid function and immune health.

- **Lifestyle Modifications**: Emily's lifestyle adjustments focus on stress reduction, sleep improvement, and exercise. Her practitioner introduces stress management techniques, including daily mindfulness exercises and deep-breathing practices to reduce cortisol levels and calm her nervous system. For sleep, she's encouraged to maintain a consistent bedtime routine, limit screen time before bed, and avoid caffeine in the afternoon. Moderate physical activity, such as yoga or brisk walking, is recommended to help reduce inflammation and improve circulation without overtaxing her system.

Together, these interventions target the underlying imbalances driving Emily's autoimmune symptoms, supporting her body's natural ability to regulate immune function and reduce inflammation.

4.1.4 Patient Outcomes and Reflection

Over the course of several months, Emily experiences noticeable improvements. Her fatigue lessens, and she reports having more energy throughout the day. Joint pain becomes less frequent, and her digestive symptoms, including bloating and irregularity, significantly decrease. Re-evaluation of her inflammatory markers shows a reduction in CRP, and her thyroid antibodies also decline, indicating less immune activity against her thyroid tissue.

Emily's case illustrates the importance of addressing root causes in managing autoimmune conditions. Rather than focusing solely on symptom suppression, her functional medicine approach tackles the underlying inflammation, gut health, and immune dysregulation fueling her symptoms. By customizing the plan to her unique genetic, lifestyle, and environmental factors, this method achieves results that traditional treatments alone may not provide. Functional medicine empowers patients to understand and manage their conditions more effectively, fostering long-term health improvements and resilience against future autoimmune flare-ups.

4.2 Metabolic Makeover: Reversing Diabetes and Metabolic Syndrome

Metabolic syndrome and type 2 diabetes are increasingly prevalent conditions characterized by high blood sugar, insulin resistance, weight gain, and fatigue. Functional medicine approaches these conditions by addressing root causes, including dietary patterns, lifestyle habits, and genetic predispositions, rather than simply managing symptoms. This case study explores how a functional medicine approach can support patients with metabolic dysfunction to regain control of their health.

4.2.1 Patient Background and Symptoms

Carlos, a 54-year-old man, has struggled with weight gain, constant fatigue, and fluctuating blood sugar levels for several years. Recently diagnosed with type 2 diabetes, he experiences frequent cravings for carbohydrates and often feels sluggish after meals. His symptoms affect his ability to perform at work and engage in physical activities, contributing to a sedentary lifestyle.

Carlos's diet consists mainly of processed foods, refined carbohydrates, and sugary snacks, which he finds convenient but acknowledges as unhealthy. Stress is another significant factor in his life, as he manages a demanding job with long hours, often turning to food for comfort. Carlos's family history includes type 2 diabetes, with both of his parents and one sibling diagnosed. His lab results indicate high fasting glucose, elevated triglycerides, low HDL cholesterol, and increased waist circumference, meeting the criteria for metabolic syndrome.

4.2.2 Functional Medicine Assessment

Carlos's functional medicine assessment uses the Functional Medicine Matrix to understand how various lifestyle, genetic, and environmental factors contribute to his metabolic dysfunction. Key areas of focus include diet, activity levels, and stress, as well as evaluating biochemical markers that indicate his metabolic health.

- **Diet and Lifestyle Factors**: Carlos's processed, high-sugar diet and lack of exercise contribute significantly to his insulin resistance and weight gain. His reliance on quick, carbohydrate-heavy snacks spikes his blood sugar, leading to energy crashes and subsequent cravings.

- **Stress and Hormones**: Chronic stress can increase cortisol levels, exacerbating blood sugar imbalances and promoting abdominal fat accumulation. Carlos's high-stress lifestyle likely plays a role in his metabolic symptoms, creating a cycle of stress-eating and further insulin resistance.

- **Genetic Predisposition**: His family history of diabetes indicates a genetic predisposition, which makes him more susceptible to metabolic dysfunction but also underscores the importance of lifestyle interventions to counteract genetic risk.

Advanced testing is essential to identify the full scope of Carlos's condition. Blood sugar monitoring reveals consistently elevated fasting glucose and HbA1c, confirming his type 2 diabetes diagnosis. Lipid panel testing shows high triglycerides and low HDL cholesterol, markers commonly associated with metabolic syndrome. Additionally, hormone testing indicates elevated cortisol, correlating with his high stress levels, while nutrient analysis reveals deficiencies in magnesium and chromium, minerals crucial for blood sugar regulation.

4.2.3 Developing the Treatment Plan

Carlos's treatment plan aims to stabilize his blood sugar, reduce inflammation, and improve his metabolic health through dietary, supplemental, and lifestyle modifications. The approach emphasizes gradual, sustainable changes that Carlos can maintain over time.

- **Dietary Changes**: Carlos is introduced to a low-glycemic, Mediterranean-style diet focused on whole foods like lean proteins, healthy fats, and fiber-rich vegetables. This diet minimizes blood sugar spikes and supports weight loss by reducing refined carbohydrates and added sugars. He receives guidance on meal planning, with an emphasis on including protein and fiber at each meal to sustain energy levels. Over time, Carlos will gradually replace sugary snacks with healthier options like nuts, seeds, and low-glycemic fruits.

- **Supplements**: Targeted supplements support Carlos's metabolic health. Chromium and magnesium are prescribed to address his deficiencies and support insulin sensitivity. Omega-3 fatty acids (from fish oil) are recommended to reduce inflammation and improve lipid profiles, while berberine, a plant compound, is included to help regulate blood sugar. Carlos is also advised to take a high-quality multivitamin to support his overall nutrient status.

- **Lifestyle Modifications**: Carlos's treatment plan incorporates stress management techniques and exercise recommendations to improve his metabolic function. Daily breathing exercises and a few minutes of mindfulness practice are introduced to help him manage stress and reduce cortisol levels. To make physical activity accessible, Carlos begins with short, brisk walks after meals to help lower post-meal blood sugar levels and gradually increases his activity as his energy improves.

- **Patient Education**: Education is central to Carlos's treatment plan. His practitioner explains the role of blood sugar stability in controlling cravings and how insulin resistance contributes to his symptoms. Carlos is encouraged to monitor his progress and set small, achievable goals, which will empower him to take ownership of his health.

4.2.4 Patient Outcomes and Reflection

Over the course of six months, Carlos experiences notable improvements. His energy levels increase, and he no longer feels drained after meals. He loses weight, particularly around his abdomen, and his blood sugar levels stabilize, as reflected in his improved HbA1c and fasting glucose measurements. Carlos's lipid profile also shows positive changes, with lower triglycerides and higher HDL cholesterol. With consistent stress management practices, he feels more balanced and better equipped to handle work-related stress without turning to food for comfort.

Carlos's case highlights the transformative power of addressing metabolic dysfunction through lifestyle and nutritional changes. Functional medicine's focus on individualized treatment allowed for a plan tailored to his specific needs, helping him make sustainable changes rather than relying solely on medications. By targeting underlying factors like diet, stress, and nutrient deficiencies, this approach provides a comprehensive solution for managing and even reversing metabolic conditions. Functional medicine enables patients like Carlos to regain control over their health, empowering them to break the cycle of metabolic dysfunction and embrace a healthier future.

4.3 Mental Health, Whole Body: Addressing Anxiety and Depression

Mental health conditions like anxiety and depression often involve a complex interplay of biological, environmental, and lifestyle factors. Traditional approaches may focus on symptom management, but functional medicine explores the underlying causes that contribute to mood instability, chronic fatigue, and disrupted sleep. By addressing factors like gut health, nutrient imbalances, and stress, functional medicine offers a holistic approach to support mental wellness. This case study illustrates how functional assessments and targeted interventions can improve mental health outcomes.

4.3.1 Patient Background and Symptoms

Sophie, a 34-year-old woman, has been struggling with chronic anxiety and intermittent depression for several years. She describes feeling "constantly on edge" and often experiences racing thoughts, irritability, and persistent fatigue. Her sleep is irregular; she has trouble falling asleep and frequently wakes up in the early hours, unable to return to rest. She also reports digestive issues, including bloating and occasional constipation, which she believes worsen when her anxiety is heightened.

Sophie's lifestyle is high-stress, with a demanding job and little time for self-care. Her diet consists mainly of processed foods and coffee, which she uses to cope with low energy throughout the day. Sophie's medical history reveals that she has been on and off various antidepressants, but with limited improvement. She has a family history of anxiety and depression, suggesting a genetic predisposition. Additionally, her diet and lifestyle likely contribute to inflammation and nutrient deficiencies, both of which can impact mood and cognitive function.

4.3.2 Functional Medicine Assessment

The functional medicine assessment for Sophie centers on identifying root causes of her anxiety and depression. The Functional Medicine Matrix is used to explore the underlying factors, including possible imbalances in the gut-brain axis, inflammation, and nutrient deficiencies.

- **Gut-Brain Axis Imbalance**: The gut-brain connection plays a crucial role in mental health, as the gut produces neurotransmitters like serotonin, which influence mood and anxiety. Sophie's digestive symptoms, such as bloating and constipation, may indicate dysbiosis or an imbalance in her gut microbiome. Poor gut health can lead to increased intestinal permeability, allowing inflammatory molecules to enter the bloodstream and potentially reach the brain, aggravating mood symptoms. A comprehensive gut health panel is recommended to assess her microbiome balance, intestinal permeability, and inflammation markers like zonulin and calprotectin.

- **Inflammation and Neurotransmitter Imbalances**: Chronic inflammation is often associated with mood disorders, as inflammatory molecules can interfere with neurotransmitter production and function. Blood tests measuring C-reactive protein (CRP) and other inflammatory markers help determine if systemic inflammation is contributing to Sophie's symptoms. Additionally, neurotransmitter testing can provide insight into levels of serotonin, dopamine, and GABA, which may be imbalanced due to chronic stress, poor diet, or genetic factors.

- **Hormone and Nutrient Deficiencies**: Hormonal imbalances, particularly involving cortisol and thyroid hormones, can affect mood, energy levels, and resilience to stress. Testing for cortisol levels throughout the day, known as a cortisol rhythm test, reveals Sophie's stress response pattern. A thyroid panel is also conducted to rule out hypothyroidism or suboptimal thyroid function, which can mimic symptoms of depression. Nutrient analysis reveals potential deficiencies in B vitamins, magnesium, and omega-3 fatty acids, all of which are essential for brain health and neurotransmitter synthesis.

4.3.3 Developing the Treatment Plan

Sophie's treatment plan focuses on supporting brain health and reducing inflammation through targeted dietary changes, supplements, and lifestyle adjustments. She begins with an anti-inflammatory diet rich in omega-3 fatty acids, essential for brain function and mood regulation. Her practitioner encourages her to incorporate foods like fatty fish, walnuts, chia seeds, and leafy greens while reducing processed foods and sugars that can contribute to inflammation. To improve her gut health, Sophie also adds fiber-rich vegetables, fermented foods like yogurt and sauerkraut, and probiotic-rich foods to support microbiome diversity.

In addition to dietary modifications, Sophie's supplementation plan includes probiotics to restore gut balance and magnesium to help regulate her sleep patterns and reduce anxiety. Omega-3 supplements, specifically EPA and DHA, are introduced to ensure she's receiving adequate anti-inflammatory support. Adaptogenic herbs like ashwagandha are recommended to help her manage stress by modulating cortisol levels. B vitamins are added to her regimen, especially B6, B9, and B12, to support neurotransmitter production and energy levels.

To address stress, her practitioner encourages daily mindfulness exercises, such as five minutes of focused breathing each morning, and suggests gentle physical activity like walking or yoga to reduce cortisol levels. Gradual habit-building in these areas allows Sophie to integrate stress reduction into her daily routine without feeling overwhelmed. This holistic approach addresses her symptoms through both biological and lifestyle adjustments, targeting the underlying factors contributing to her anxiety and depression.

4.3.4 Patient Outcomes and Reflection

Over the course of three months, Sophie reports significant improvements in her mood, energy, and sleep quality. She experiences fewer episodes of anxiety and feels a greater sense of calm, even during stressful periods. Her sleep becomes more consistent, with fewer early-morning awakenings, allowing her to wake up refreshed. Digestive symptoms, such as bloating and irregular bowel movements, also decrease, contributing to a better sense of overall well-being. Blood tests reveal reductions in inflammatory markers, and follow-up testing shows improvements in her microbiome diversity and cortisol levels.

Sophie's case highlights the profound connection between mental health and physical health. Addressing underlying issues in her gut, managing inflammation, and supporting neurotransmitter balance led to positive shifts in her mental well-being. This functional medicine approach goes beyond symptom management, treating the root causes of her anxiety and depression and providing a comprehensive, sustainable path to improved mental health.

Key Takeaways

Functional medicine assessments reveal underlying causes of complex conditions. Personalized treatment plans can address chronic issues effectively. Real-life cases illustrate how nurse practitioners can apply these methods in practice.

Think about patients in your practice who might benefit from a root-cause analysis. Consider which functional assessment tools and lifestyle recommendations could be integrated into patient care. In the next chapter, explore strategies for incorporating functional medicine into a busy practice.

Chapter 5: Building Your Practice: Integrating Functional Medicine in Real-World Settings

"In order to change the world, you have to get your head together first."
– Jimi Hendrix

Emily, a nurse practitioner passionate about functional medicine, quickly found herself overwhelmed when she began implementing it in her busy practice. Her intention was to provide root-cause-focused care, yet time constraints, extensive documentation, and administrative demands threatened to derail her efforts. Patients appreciated the depth of her approach, but Emily found it nearly impossible to balance thorough assessments with the fast-paced demands of her clinic.

After much trial and error, she discovered strategies that allowed her to make functional medicine practical and sustainable. By restructuring her workflow, integrating technology, and streamlining her documentation, Emily transformed her practice. She was able to provide high-quality care without sacrificing efficiency or compassion.

This chapter focuses on practical strategies for integrating functional medicine into a typical clinical setting. You'll learn how to create a structured workflow, manage documentation and compliance effectively, and maintain patient-centered communication. With these tools, functional medicine can become a feasible, rewarding part of your practice, empowering you to offer deeper, more meaningful care.

5.1 Creating a Functional Medicine Workflow: Efficiency Meets Empathy

Integrating functional medicine into a conventional practice setting comes with unique workflow challenges. Nurse practitioners often encounter limited appointment times, a high patient load, and extensive administrative tasks, which can make providing thorough, root-cause-focused care difficult. Functional medicine assessments typically require more time and detail than standard visits, involving extensive history-taking, dietary guidance, and lifestyle modifications. Additionally, managing follow-ups and documenting complex treatment plans can become overwhelming without a structured approach. By building an efficient workflow tailored to functional medicine's demands, nurse practitioners can overcome these challenges while maintaining a high standard of patient-centered care.

Developing a Step-by-Step Functional Medicine Workflow

An efficient functional medicine workflow supports comprehensive patient care without compromising productivity. Here is a step-by-step guide for creating a workflow that balances thorough assessments with time management.

1. **Initial Patient Assessment**

The initial assessment is foundational in functional medicine, as it sets the stage for understanding each patient's unique health needs. Schedule these first appointments with additional time (ideally 60-90 minutes) to cover a comprehensive intake. Use pre-visit questionnaires and intake forms to gather essential information before the appointment. This not only prepares you but also allows patients to reflect on their symptoms, lifestyle, and medical history in advance. Focus on identifying antecedents, triggers, and mediators, following the Functional Medicine Matrix as a framework.

2. **Follow-Up Appointments**

Consistent follow-ups are essential for tracking patient progress and adjusting treatment plans as needed. For efficiency, schedule shorter follow-ups (20-30 minutes) after the initial intake, with specific goals in mind—such as reviewing dietary changes, monitoring symptom progression, or discussing test results. Follow-ups can be scheduled at different intervals based on each patient's needs, with more frequent check-ins in the beginning and less frequent visits as they achieve stability.

3. **Case Review and Planning**

Allocate dedicated time each week for case review and treatment planning. This allows you to revisit complex cases, assess patient progress, and update treatment plans in an organized manner. Group similar cases for more efficient planning, focusing on patients with overlapping needs (e.g., gut health or metabolic concerns). Weekly planning also prevents last-minute decision-making and ensures you remain proactive rather than reactive in patient care.

Using Technology to Streamline Workflow

Technology plays a crucial role in making functional medicine workflows more efficient. Implementing the right tools can reduce administrative burdens and facilitate better patient tracking.

- **Electronic Health Records (EHR) Systems**: EHRs designed for integrative and functional medicine can simplify documentation, making it easier to record complex data, track symptom progression, and manage treatment plans. Functional medicine EHRs often come with customizable templates that streamline data entry, focusing on the Functional Medicine Matrix and symptom patterns.

- **Symptom-Tracking Apps**: Encourage patients to use symptom-tracking apps, which allow them to monitor their progress between visits. These apps enable patients to log symptoms, dietary intake, and lifestyle changes, providing you with real-time data that aids in more precise treatment adjustments. Reviewing these logs during follow-ups can offer quick insights and allow for targeted interventions.

- **Digital Patient Education Resources**: Digital resources, like patient portals and educational videos, empower patients to engage with their treatment outside of appointments. Educational materials on nutrition, lifestyle changes, and supplement use can be shared through a secure portal, helping patients better understand and adhere to their care plans. This approach also reduces the need for repeated explanations, saving time during appointments.

Maintaining Empathy in a Busy Schedule

Efficiency doesn't mean sacrificing empathy. In functional medicine, a patient-centered approach is crucial to fostering trust and engagement, both of which contribute to better outcomes. Here are a few ways to maintain empathy in a fast-paced environment:

- **Active Listening**: Take a few moments to listen actively during each visit, acknowledging the patient's concerns and validating their experiences. Active listening doesn't have to be time-consuming, but it demonstrates that you're fully present and invested in their health.

- **Compassionate Communication**: Explain your recommendations clearly and empathetically. Functional medicine often involves significant lifestyle changes, which can feel overwhelming. Show empathy by acknowledging the challenges patients may face and offering encouragement and support as they implement these changes.

- **Ensuring Patients Feel Valued**: Simple gestures, such as using their name, summarizing key points to show you've listened, and setting collaborative goals, go a long way in making patients feel valued and understood. When patients feel respected, they are more likely to adhere to their treatment plans.

Case Example

Dr. Lopez, a nurse practitioner with a busy integrative care practice, found herself struggling to balance functional medicine assessments with her patient load. Initially, she felt rushed during visits, which affected her ability to provide the level of care she wanted. After implementing a structured workflow, she saw immediate improvements. She began by extending initial consultations to 90 minutes, using pre-visit questionnaires to gather background information in advance. For follow-ups, she adopted a consistent structure, with specific goals for each appointment, like reviewing dietary logs or addressing a single symptom.

Dr. Lopez also introduced technology into her practice. She selected an EHR tailored to functional medicine, which enabled her to document efficiently and review each patient's Functional Medicine Matrix at a glance. Her patients used symptom-tracking apps to log daily changes, allowing her to quickly assess progress during follow-ups. She also created a library of digital resources covering topics like anti-inflammatory diets, supplement protocols, and relaxation techniques, which patients accessed through a secure portal.

This approach not only improved her efficiency but also allowed her to maintain empathy. By reducing administrative tasks, Dr. Lopez had more time to engage with her patients directly. During appointments, she practiced active listening and collaborated on setting achievable goals. Over time, she found that patients were more engaged, treatment adherence improved, and her practice ran more smoothly, embodying functional medicine's balance of efficiency and empathy.

5.2 Documentation and Compliance: Navigating Insurance and Legalities

Thorough documentation is essential in functional medicine, especially when managing complex, multi-systemic health issues. Functional medicine visits often involve detailed patient histories, comprehensive assessments, and personalized treatment plans. Accurate and thorough documentation not only supports better patient outcomes but also safeguards nurse practitioners legally. Clear records provide a transparent view of patient care, allowing for continuity across visits and ensuring all aspects of the patient's health journey are documented. Additionally, thorough documentation establishes a legal record that demonstrates adherence to best practices, protecting the practitioner in case of audits or legal challenges.

Best Practices for Documentation

Effective documentation in functional medicine requires attention to detail, especially in capturing the holistic approach of this model. Here are key practices to ensure accurate and organized records:

- **Detailing Patient History and Assessment**: The Functional Medicine Matrix is a critical tool for organizing patient data. Documenting antecedents, triggers, and mediators provides a comprehensive overview of the factors contributing to the patient's condition. For instance, noting a patient's history of antibiotic use (an antecedent) may correlate with gut health issues, while identifying high-stress levels as a trigger could point to inflammation or immune dysregulation. Documenting this layered information enables a clearer understanding of the root causes, supporting a more targeted treatment approach.

- **Treatment Plans and Progress Notes**: Functional medicine treatment plans often include dietary adjustments, supplement protocols, and lifestyle modifications, all of which need to be documented clearly. Each component of the plan should be recorded, with details on dosages for supplements, frequency for lifestyle practices, and specific dietary recommendations. Progress notes should capture patient responses to the plan, including any symptom changes and adjustments made during follow-ups, creating a continuous record of patient progress.

- **Using Templates and Forms**: Pre-made templates for functional medicine visits streamline documentation, ensuring consistency across appointments. Templates can prompt practitioners to record each section of the Functional Medicine Matrix, note lab results, and list treatment recommendations. This approach saves time while helping to maintain thorough records, even with a high patient load.

Insurance Coding and Billing in Functional Medicine

Navigating insurance billing can be challenging in functional medicine, as certain assessments and treatments may not align with traditional models. Using the right codes and effectively communicating with patients about costs are essential for a sustainable practice.

- **Common CPT Codes**: Functional medicine visits often require codes that reflect extended consultations and complex assessments. Commonly used CPT codes include 99204 or 99205 for initial evaluations, which cover comprehensive assessments. For follow-up visits, codes like 99213 or 99214 may apply, depending on the complexity and time required.

- **Billing for Extended Time**: Functional medicine appointments, particularly initial assessments, often exceed standard timeframes. When possible, bill for extended time using prolonged services codes like 99354, which apply to sessions lasting beyond typical durations. Billing for the actual time spent allows practitioners to receive fair compensation for in-depth assessments and follow-ups.

- **Educating Patients on Out-of-Pocket Costs**: Insurance may not cover all aspects of a functional medicine visit, especially tests and supplements. It's crucial to communicate anticipated costs with patients upfront, explaining the value of the services offered. Emphasize that these investments support comprehensive care, targeting root causes rather than just symptom management, and encourage patients to weigh the benefits of this approach.

Legal Considerations and Compliance

Ensuring legal compliance is essential for functional medicine practitioners. Here are some key considerations:

- **Scope of Practice**: Nurse practitioners should operate within their licensed scope, following both state and national guidelines. Certain treatments may require specific certifications or collaborative agreements with other healthcare providers. Adhering to scope of practice guidelines not only ensures patient safety but also prevents potential legal issues.

- **HIPAA and Patient Confidentiality**: Patient confidentiality is paramount, especially with the sensitive nature of functional medicine assessments, which often explore lifestyle and personal health details. Use HIPAA-compliant electronic systems to safeguard patient records, and maintain strict confidentiality in communications with patients and other healthcare providers.

- **Informed Consent**: Functional medicine may involve non-standard treatments, such as specific supplements or lifestyle recommendations. Obtaining informed consent is critical when introducing these interventions. Discuss the risks and benefits of each recommended treatment, and document these conversations in the patient's record. Informed consent not only protects patients but also provides a legal safeguard for practitioners.

Case Example

Dr. Martin, a nurse practitioner specializing in functional medicine, worked with a patient, Sarah, who had chronic digestive issues and fatigue. To get to the root of her symptoms, Dr. Martin conducted a comprehensive assessment, including advanced testing and dietary recommendations that were outside conventional protocols. Throughout Sarah's treatment, Dr. Martin meticulously documented each step: the Functional Medicine Matrix, treatment plan, and progress notes detailing symptom changes and dietary adjustments.

For billing, Dr. Martin used extended time codes due to the complexity of Sarah's case, ensuring appropriate compensation for the extended consultations. She also discussed potential out-of-pocket costs for specific tests, helping Sarah understand the value and expected outcomes. When Sarah's insurance provider requested additional details during an audit, Dr. Martin's organized records provided a clear view of the medically necessary services, supporting her decisions and securing reimbursement.

This case illustrates the importance of documentation, compliance, and patient communication in functional medicine. Dr. Martin's thorough documentation not only protected her practice but also enhanced Sarah's treatment experience by fostering transparency and trust.

Key Takeaways

A structured workflow enables efficient integration of functional medicine. Thorough documentation and adherence to insurance and legal guidelines are essential for effective, compliant practice. Patient-centered communication and empathy foster adherence and satisfaction, enhancing outcomes in functional medicine.

Begin developing a functional medicine workflow suited to your practice. Review documentation practices to meet functional medicine standards and explore tech tools to improve efficiency. In the final chapter, we'll focus on empowering patients for sustainable, long-term health success.

Conclusion

"The physician treats, but nature heals."
– Hippocrates

Adopting a functional medicine approach represents a meaningful shift for nurse practitioners, one that redefines patient care by focusing on root causes and comprehensive wellness. This book has guided you through the essential aspects of functional medicine, offering a framework for delivering personalized, patient-centered care that addresses the underlying factors driving health issues. As you reflect on the journey presented in these pages, recognize the transformative impact functional medicine can have on your practice and the fulfillment that comes from helping patients achieve lasting health improvements.

Throughout this book, we explored a comprehensive approach to integrating functional medicine into your practice. The introduction provided an overview of functional medicine's potential to transform nurse practitioner care by moving beyond symptom management to root-cause solutions. Chapter 1 highlighted the limitations of conventional symptom-based treatment and the benefits of adopting a functional approach focused on understanding and addressing root causes.

In Chapter 2, we examined patient-centered assessment tools, such as the Functional Medicine Matrix and thorough history-taking, which allow you to understand each patient's unique health profile fully. Chapter 3 introduced core functional medicine interventions, emphasizing the critical role of nutrition, supplements, and lifestyle adjustments. Real-life case studies in Chapter 4 illustrated how these principles apply to common, complex conditions like autoimmune disorders, metabolic syndrome, and mental health challenges, providing practical examples for integrating functional medicine in clinical settings. Finally, Chapter 5 addressed practical strategies for implementing functional medicine, from creating efficient workflows to navigating documentation and compliance, offering the tools you need to integrate this approach seamlessly into your practice.

The core message throughout this book is that functional medicine empowers nurse practitioners to practice a deeper, holistic level of care. By treating patients as whole individuals rather than isolated symptoms, you foster a collaborative approach that empowers both you and your patients to work toward sustained health and wellness.

To begin implementing functional medicine principles immediately, consider reviewing patient cases in your current practice. Look for patterns in their symptoms or lifestyle factors that might indicate underlying root causes and think about how functional medicine's tools—such as dietary modifications or stress management strategies—could make a difference in their care.

For ongoing professional development, explore resources like online courses, functional medicine certifications, and relevant conferences. Joining a community of functional medicine practitioners can provide support, insights, and shared learning experiences that enrich your practice and broaden your perspective.

As you move forward, view yourself as a change agent in healthcare, bridging gaps in traditional treatment models and setting new standards in patient-centered care. Functional medicine enables you to deliver comprehensive wellness by focusing on the foundational aspects of health, from nutrition and lifestyle to mind-body balance.

Carry the insights and practices from this book into each patient interaction, building trust, and fostering long-term health improvements. Embrace functional medicine as a powerful tool for creating transformative patient care and continue leading the way in a healthcare approach that not only treats but also empowers.

www.ingramcontent.com/pod-product-compliance
Lightning Source LLC
Chambersburg PA
CBHW050254220526
45465CB00002B/682